THE CANDIDA CLEANSE DIET COOKBOOK

Dr. Kimberly Carlos

Copyright © 2023 by Dr. Kimberly Carlos

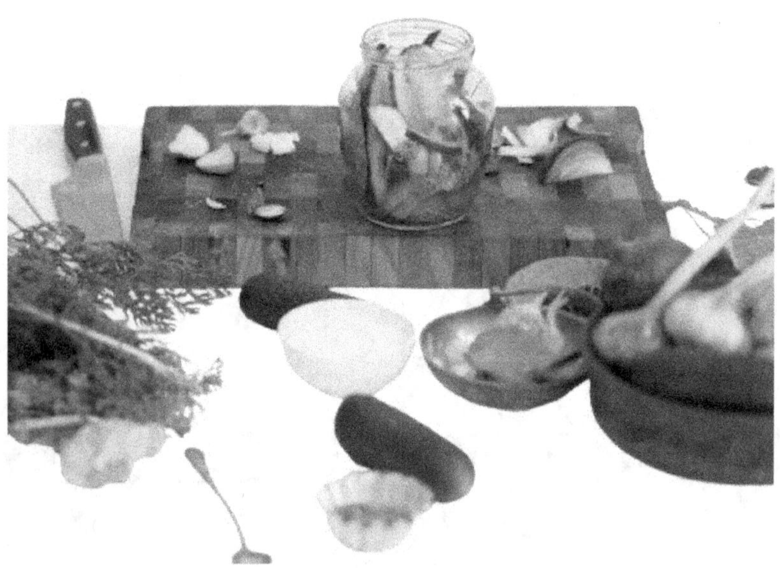

TABLE OF CONTENT

CHAPTER ONE

Types, Causes and Symptoms of Candida

Candida is a type of yeast or fungus that naturally resides in our bodies, primarily in the gut and mucous membranes. In normal circumstances, it coexists harmlessly with other microorganisms, but when the balance is disrupted, it can lead to various types of infections.

There are different types of candida, each with its own set of causes and symptoms. Below, we'll explore the most common types of candida infections, their potential causes, and the associated symptoms:

1. Candidiasis (Thrush):

- **Type:** Oral Candidiasis (Thrush)
- **Cause:** Weakened immune system, antibiotics, steroid use, or poor oral hygiene.
- **Symptoms:** White or yellow patches in the mouth, tongue, and throat, along with pain, difficulty swallowing, and altered taste sensation.

2. Vaginal Candidiasis (Vaginal Yeast Infection):

- **Type:** Vaginal Candidiasis
- **Cause:** Hormonal changes (pregnancy, menopause), antibiotic use, uncontrolled diabetes, or a weakened immune system.
- **Symptoms:** Itching, burning, redness, swelling, and white, curd-like vaginal discharge.

3. Cutaneous Candidiasis:

- **Type:** Cutaneous Candidiasis
- **Cause:** Warm and moist skin environments, such as skin folds, can create ideal conditions for candida overgrowth.
- **Symptoms:** Red, itchy rash with well-defined borders, often found in skin folds like armpits, groin, and beneath the breasts.

4. Invasive Candidiasis:

- **Type:** Invasive Candidiasis
- **Cause:** Typically occurs in hospitalized patients with weakened immune systems, indwelling catheters, or recent surgery.

- **Symptoms:** Varies depending on the affected organ but may include fever, chills, low blood pressure, and organ dysfunction.

5. Chronic Mucocutaneous Candidiasis (CMC):

- **Type:** Chronic Mucocutaneous Candidiasis
- **Cause:** Genetic predisposition, immune system disorders.
- **Symptoms:** Frequent and recurring candida infections affecting mucous membranes, skin, and nails, leading to discomfort and persistent rashes.

6. Systemic Candidiasis:

- **Type:** Systemic Candidiasis
- **Cause:** Severe immunosuppression or organ transplantation.
- **Symptoms:** Serious systemic infection with fever, chills, fatigue, and organ dysfunction. It can be life-threatening.

How to Follow a Candida Cleansing Diet with Its Benefits

Following a candida cleansing diet can be beneficial for those dealing with candida overgrowth or fungal infections. The diet aims to starve the candida fungus by eliminating the foods it thrives on while promoting the growth of beneficial gut bacteria. Here's a guide on how to follow a candida cleansing diet with its associated benefits:

1. Eliminate Candida-Friendly Foods

- **Sugars:** Avoid all forms of sugar, including refined sugars, high-fructose corn syrup, and even natural sugars like honey and maple syrup.
- **Refined Carbohydrates:** Stay away from white bread, pasta, and processed foods, as these quickly convert to sugar in the body.
- **Processed Foods:** Eliminate processed and packaged foods that may contain hidden sugars and additives.
- **Alcohol:** Alcohol can feed candida, so it's best to avoid it during the cleansing period.

2. Focus on Whole, Unprocessed Foods:

- **Non-Starchy Vegetables:** Load up on leafy greens, broccoli, cauliflower, zucchini, and other non-starchy vegetables.
- **Lean Proteins:** Include sources like chicken, fish, turkey, and tofu.
- **Healthy Fats:** Opt for sources such as avocados, nuts, seeds, and olive oil.

3. Incorporate Antifungal Foods:

- **Garlic:** Garlic has natural antifungal properties, so use it liberally in your meals.
- **Coconut Oil:** Coconut oil contains caprylic acid, which is known to combat candida.
- **Ginger and Turmeric:** These spices have anti-inflammatory and antifungal properties.

4. Eat Probiotic-Rich Foods:

- **Yogurt:** Choose unsweetened, plain yogurt with live cultures or dairy-free alternatives like coconut yogurt.
- **Kefir:** This fermented dairy or non-dairy drink is rich in probiotics.

- **Sauerkraut, Kimchi, and Fermented Pickles**: These foods promote a healthy gut microbiome.

5. Stay Hydrated: Drink plenty of water to help flush toxins from your system.

6. Limit Dairy: Dairy products can sometimes exacerbate candida symptoms, so consider reducing or eliminating them.

7. Plan Balanced Meals: Create balanced meals that combine protein, healthy fats, and non-starchy vegetables to help stabilize blood sugar levels.

Benefits of a Candida Cleansing Diet

1. Symptom Relief: Many people report relief from candida-related symptoms like digestive issues, skin problems, and fatigue.

2. Balanced Gut Microbiome: The diet can promote the growth of beneficial gut bacteria, which is crucial for overall health.

3. Weight Management: Eliminating sugar and refined carbs can aid in weight management and stabilize blood sugar levels.

4. Improved Immunity: A healthy gut contributes to a stronger immune system.

5. Long-Term Health: By adopting a diet focused on whole, unprocessed foods, you may establish healthier eating habits that benefit your long-term well-being.

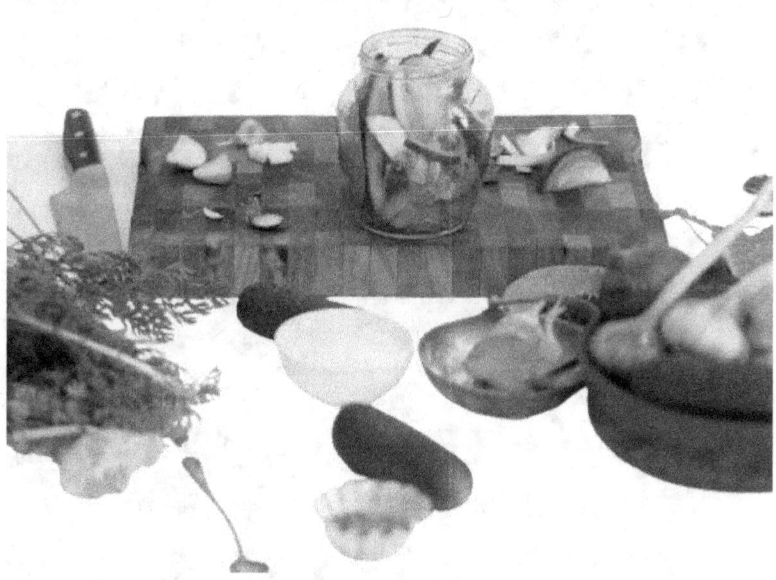

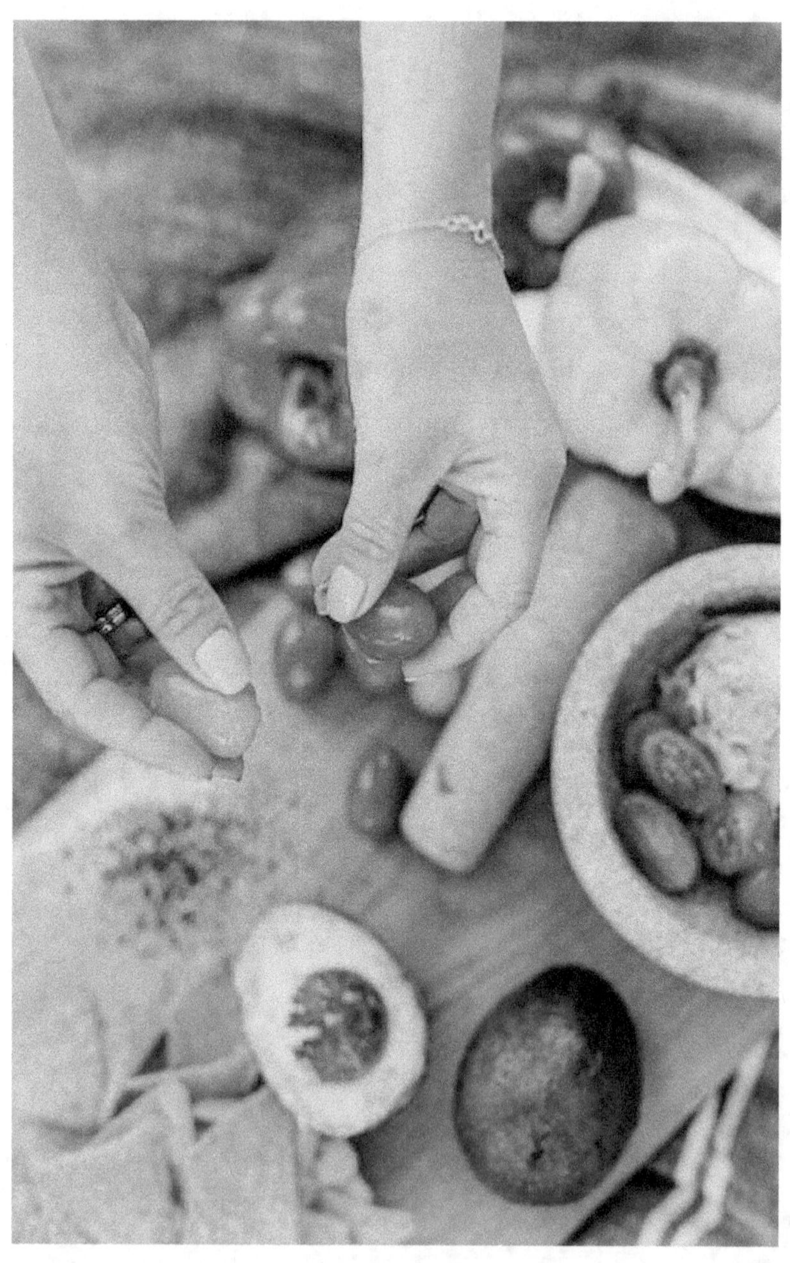

CHAPTER TWO

14-Day Candida Cleansing Diet Meal Plan

A 14-day candida cleansing diet meal plan focuses on eliminating candida-feeding foods while incorporating anti-fungal and gut-friendly options. Here's a sample meal plan to get you started:

Day 1

- Breakfast: Scrambled eggs with spinach and a side of sautéed mushrooms.
- Lunch: Grilled chicken breast salad with mixed greens, cucumber, and homemade vinaigrette.
- Snack: Carrot and celery sticks with almond butter.
- Dinner: Baked salmon with steamed broccoli and a side of quinoa.

Day 2

- **Breakfast:** Greek yogurt with a handful of fresh berries.
- **Lunch:** Lentil soup with a side of mixed greens.
- **Snack:** Sliced bell peppers with hummus.
- Dinner: Grilled shrimp with asparagus and cauliflower rice.

Day 3

- **Breakfast:** Smoothie with spinach, avocado, coconut milk, and a scoop of protein powder.
- **Lunch:** Tuna salad with mixed greens and a lemon-tahini dressing.
- **Snack:** A small serving of unsweetened coconut yogurt.
- **Dinner:** Roasted chicken with Brussels sprouts and a side of quinoa.

Day 4

- **Breakfast:** Omelet with sautéed spinach, tomatoes, and feta cheese.
- **Lunch:** Turkey and avocado lettuce wraps with a side of fermented sauerkraut.
- **Snack:** Cucumber slices with guacamole.
- **Dinner:** Baked cod with roasted asparagus and a side of mashed cauliflower.

Day 5

- **Breakfast:** Chia seed pudding with almond milk and topped with sliced strawberries.
- **Lunch:** Spinach and kale salad with grilled tofu and a

balsamic vinaigrette.

- **Snack:** A handful of mixed nuts (unsalted).
- **Dinner:** Beef stir-fry with broccoli, bell peppers, and garlic in a coconut aminos sauce.

Day 6

- **Breakfast:** Cottage cheese with sliced peaches and a sprinkle of cinnamon.
- **Lunch:** Quinoa and black bean salad with diced tomatoes, corn, and cilantro.
- **Snack:** Sliced apple with a small serving of almond butter.
- **Dinner:** Baked chicken thighs with steamed green beans and a side of brown rice.

Day 7

- **Breakfast:** Smoothie with kale, banana, almond milk, and a spoon of almond butter.
- **Lunch:** Zucchini noodles with pesto sauce and grilled shrimp.
- **Snack:** Celery sticks with sunflower seed butter.
- **Dinner:** Roasted turkey with roasted Brussels sprouts and a side of mashed sweet potatoes.

Day 8

- **Breakfast:** Scrambled eggs with sautéed spinach and a side of sliced avocado.
- **Lunch:** Grilled chicken breast with steamed broccoli and a quinoa salad with chopped cucumber and parsley.
- **Snack:** Sliced bell peppers with tzatziki sauce.
- **Dinner:** Baked salmon with roasted asparagus and a side of mashed cauliflower.

Day 9

- **Breakfast:** A smoothie with kale, banana, coconut milk, and a scoop of plant-based protein powder.
- **Lunch:** Tuna and avocado lettuce wraps with a side of fermented kimchi.
- **Snack:** Sliced cucumber with guacamole.
- **Dinner:** Grilled shrimp with sautéed kale and brown rice.

Day 10

- **Breakfast:** Greek yogurt with sliced strawberries and a drizzle of honey (if desired).
- **Lunch:** Lentil soup with a side of mixed greens and a

lemon-tahini dressing.

- **Snack:** A small serving of unsweetened coconut yogurt.
- **Dinner:** Baked chicken thighs with roasted Brussels sprouts and a side of quinoa.

Day 11

- **Breakfast:** Omelet with diced tomatoes, bell peppers, and feta cheese.
- **Lunch:** Turkey and avocado lettuce wraps with a side of fermented sauerkraut.
- **Snack:** Carrot and celery sticks with almond butter.
- **Dinner:** Beef stir-fry with broccoli, cauliflower, and garlic in a coconut aminos sauce.

Day 12

- **Breakfast:** Chia seed pudding with almond milk and topped with fresh blueberries.
- **Lunch:** Spinach and kale salad with grilled tofu and a balsamic vinaigrette.
- **Snack:** A handful of mixed nuts (unsalted).
- **Dinner:** Baked cod with steamed green beans and a side of mashed sweet potatoes.

Day 13

- Breakfast: Cottage cheese with sliced peaches and a sprinkle of cinnamon.
- Lunch: Quinoa and black bean salad with diced tomatoes, corn, and cilantro.
- Snack: Sliced apple with a small serving of almond butter.
- Dinner: Roasted turkey with roasted asparagus and a side of cauliflower rice.

Day 14

- Breakfast: Smoothie with spinach, banana, almond milk, and a spoon of almond butter.
- Lunch: Zucchini noodles with pesto sauce and grilled shrimp.
- Snack: Sliced pear with a dollop of coconut yogurt.
- Dinner: Grilled chicken breast with sautéed spinach and a side of brown rice.

CHAPTER THREE

Candida Cleansing Breakfast Recipes

Starting your day with a candida cleansing breakfast sets the tone for a day of balanced nutrition. These breakfast recipes are designed to be delicious, satisfying, and free of candida-promoting ingredients, helping you maintain a healthy gut and combat candida overgrowth.

1. Avocado and Poached Eggs on Almond Toast

Ingredients:

- 2 eggs
- 1 ripe avocado
- 2 slices of almond bread
- Salt and pepper to taste
- Fresh herbs for garnish (optional)

Instructions:

1. Poach the eggs to your preferred level of doneness.

2. While the eggs are poaching, toast the almond bread until lightly crispy.

3. Mash the ripe avocado and spread it on the toasted almond

bread.

4. Place the poached eggs on top of the avocado.

5. Season with salt, pepper, and garnish with fresh herbs if desired.

Cooking Time: 15 minutes.

2. Greek Yogurt Parfait with Berries

Ingredients:

- 1 cup of Greek yogurt (unsweetened)
- A handful of mixed berries (e.g., blueberries, strawberries, raspberries)
- 2 tablespoons of chia seeds
- A drizzle of honey (optional)
- Chopped nuts for crunch (optional)

Instructions:

1. In a bowl or glass, layer Greek yogurt, mixed berries, and chia seeds.

2. Repeat the layers until the container is filled.

3. Drizzle honey on top for sweetness if desired.

4. Top with chopped nuts for added texture.

Cooking Time: 5 minutes (if you've prepped the chia seeds in advance).

3. Spinach and Mushroom Omelet

Ingredients:

-   2 eggs
-   Handful of spinach leaves
-   1/4 cup sliced mushrooms
-   1/4 cup diced onions
-   Salt and pepper to taste
-   Olive oil for cooking

Instructions:

1. Heat olive oil in a pan over medium heat.

2. Add diced onions and sliced mushrooms. Sauté until they become tender.

3. Add spinach leaves and cook until wilted.

4. Whisk eggs in a bowl and pour them into the pan over the vegetables.

5. Cook until the omelet is set, then fold it in half.

6. Season with salt and pepper before serving.

Cooking Time: 10 minutes.

4. Coconut Chia Pudding

Ingredients:

- 3 tablespoons chia seeds
- 1 cup unsweetened coconut milk
- 1/2 teaspoon pure vanilla extract
- A drizzle of honey (optional)
- Fresh berries for topping

Instructions:

1. In a bowl, mix chia seeds, coconut milk, and vanilla extract.

2. Stir well and let it sit in the refrigerator for at least 3 hours or overnight.

3. Before serving, sweeten with honey if desired and top with fresh berries.

Cooking Time: 3 hours (mostly resting time).

5. Almond Butter and Banana Smoothie

Ingredients:

- 1 ripe banana
- 2 tablespoons almond butter
- 1 cup almond milk (unsweetened)
- 1/2 teaspoon cinnamon
- A drizzle of honey (optional)
- Ice cubes (optional)

Instructions:

1. Combine the banana, almond butter, almond milk, cinnamon, and honey (if using) in a blender.

2. Blend until smooth.

3. Add ice cubes and blend again for a colder, creamier texture.

Cooking Time: 5 minutes.

6. Quinoa Breakfast Bowl

Ingredients:

- 1/2 cup cooked quinoa

- 1/4 cup unsweetened Greek yogurt

- Sliced almonds

- Fresh berries (e.g., strawberries, blueberries)

- A drizzle of honey (optional)

Instructions:

1. In a bowl, layer cooked quinoa, Greek yogurt, and fresh berries.

2. Top with sliced almonds and drizzle honey for sweetness if desired.

Cooking Time: 5 minutes (if quinoa is pre-cooked).

7. Spinach and Mushroom Breakfast Wrap

Ingredients:

- 2 large collard green leaves (for wrapping)

- Scrambled eggs

- Sautéed spinach and mushrooms (similar to recipe #3)

- Avocado slices

- Salsa or hot sauce (optional)

Instructions:

1. Lay the collard green leaves flat.

2. Layer scrambled eggs, sautéed spinach and mushrooms, avocado slices, and salsa (if desired).

3. Roll up the collard leaves like a burrito, tucking in the sides.

Cooking Time: 15 minutes (including sautéing).

8. Apple Cinnamon Oatmeal

Ingredients:

- 1/2 cup gluten-free rolled oats
- 1 cup unsweetened almond milk
- 1 apple, diced
- 1/2 teaspoon cinnamon
- Chopped nuts (e.g., walnuts or almonds)
- A drizzle of honey (optional)

Instructions:

1. In a saucepan, combine oats, almond milk, diced apple, and cinnamon.

2. Cook on low heat, stirring occasionally, until the oats are creamy and the apple is tender.

3. Serve with chopped nuts and honey if desired.

Cooking Time: 10-15 minutes.

9. Sweet Potato Hash

Ingredients:

- 1 sweet potato, diced
- 1/4 cup diced bell peppers
- 1/4 cup diced onions
- 1/4 cup diced zucchini
- 1/4 teaspoon paprika
- Olive oil for cooking
- Fresh parsley for garnish (optional)

Instructions:

1. Heat olive oil in a pan over medium heat.

2. Add diced sweet potatoes and sauté until they start to brown and soften.

3. Add bell peppers, onions, and zucchini. Sauté until all the

vegetables are tender.

4. Season with paprika and garnish with fresh parsley if desired.

Cooking Time: 15 minutes.

10. Almond Flour Pancakes

Ingredients:

- 1 cup almond flour
- 2 eggs
- 1/4 cup unsweetened almond milk
- 1/2 teaspoon baking soda
- A pinch of salt
- Coconut oil for cooking
- Fresh berries for topping
- A drizzle of honey (optional)

Instructions:

1. In a bowl, whisk together almond flour, eggs, almond milk, baking soda, and a pinch of salt until you have a smooth batter.

2. Heat coconut oil in a skillet over medium heat.

3. Pour small portions of the batter onto the skillet to make pancakes.

4. Cook until bubbles form on the surface, then flip and cook until both sides are golden brown.

5. Top with fresh berries and a drizzle of honey if desired.

Cooking Time: 15 minutes.

Candida Cleansing Lunch Recipes

Lunch can be a satisfying and nutritious part of your candida cleansing journey. These lunch recipes are free of candida-promoting ingredients and focus on whole, unprocessed foods to support your digestive health.

1. Quinoa and Vegetable Stir-Fry

Ingredients:

- 1 cup cooked quinoa
- Assorted vegetables (bell peppers, broccoli, carrots, snap peas)
- Garlic and ginger (minced)
- Coconut aminos (for seasoning)
- Olive oil for stir-frying

- Fresh cilantro for garnish (optional)

Instructions:

1. Heat olive oil in a pan.

2. Sauté minced garlic and ginger until fragrant.

3. Add assorted vegetables and stir-fry until tender.

4. Stir in cooked quinoa and season with coconut aminos.

5. Garnish with fresh cilantro if desired.

Cooking Time: 15-20 minutes.

2. Lentil and Vegetable Soup

Ingredients:

- 1 cup cooked lentils
- Assorted vegetables (carrots, celery, onion, spinach)
- Vegetable broth
- Garlic (minced)
- Cumin and paprika (for seasoning)
- Olive oil for sautéing

Instructions:

1. Heat olive oil in a pot and sauté minced garlic.

2. Add chopped vegetables and cook until they start to soften.

3. Stir in cooked lentils and vegetable broth.

4. Season with cumin and paprika.

5. Simmer until the vegetables are tender.

Cooking Time: 30-40 minutes.

3. Grilled Chicken and Avocado Salad

Ingredients:

- Grilled chicken breast
- Mixed greens (e.g., lettuce, spinach)
- Sliced cucumber and cherry tomatoes
- Sliced avocado
- Olive oil and lemon juice (for dressing)

Instructions:

1. Grill the chicken until fully cooked.

2. In a bowl, combine mixed greens, cucumber, cherry

tomatoes, and sliced avocado.

3. Slice the grilled chicken and add it to the salad.

4. Drizzle with olive oil and lemon juice for dressing.

Cooking Time: Depends on chicken grilling time.

4. Baked Salmon with Steamed Vegetables

Ingredients:

- Salmon fillet
- Assorted vegetables (e.g., broccoli, cauliflower, carrots)
- Olive oil, lemon, and dill (for seasoning)

Instructions:

1. Season the salmon with olive oil, lemon juice, and dill.

2. Bake the salmon in the oven until it flakes easily.

3. Steam the assorted vegetables until tender.

4. Serve the salmon with steamed vegetables on the side.

Cooking Time: 15-20 minutes.

5. Zucchini Noodles with Pesto and Cherry Tomatoes

Ingredients:

- Zucchini noodles (zoodles)
- Pesto sauce (make sure it's candida-friendly)
- Cherry tomatoes (halved)
- Pine nuts (toasted, optional)

Instructions:

1. Spiralize the zucchini to make noodles.

2. In a pan, lightly sauté the zoodles until tender.

3. Toss the zoodles with pesto sauce and halved cherry tomatoes.

4. Top with toasted pine nuts if desired.

Cooking Time: 10 minutes.

6. Turkey and Avocado Lettuce Wraps

Ingredients:

- Ground turkey
- Romaine lettuce leaves

- Sliced avocado

- Salsa (make sure it's candida-friendly)

Instructions:

1. Cook ground turkey in a skillet until browned and cooked through.

2. Place a scoop of cooked turkey on a romaine lettuce leaf.

3. Top with sliced avocado and salsa.

4. Roll up the lettuce leaf and enjoy.

Cooking Time: 15 minutes.

7. Cauliflower Rice Stir-Fry

Ingredients:

- Cauliflower rice
- Mixed vegetables (e.g., bell peppers, snap peas, carrots)
- Garlic and ginger (minced)
- Coconut aminos (for seasoning)
- Olive oil for stir-frying

Instructions:

1. Heat olive oil in a pan.

2. Sauté minced garlic and ginger until fragrant.

3. Add mixed vegetables and stir-fry until tender.

4. Stir in cauliflower rice and season with coconut aminos.

5. Cook until the cauliflower rice is heated through.

Cooking Time: 15-20 minutes.

8. Chickpea and Spinach Salad

Ingredients:

- Cooked chickpeas
- Fresh spinach leaves
- Diced cucumber and red onion
- Lemon-tahini dressing (candida-friendly)
- Fresh parsley for garnish (optional)

Instructions:

1. In a bowl, combine chickpeas, spinach, cucumber, and red onion.

2. Drizzle with lemon-tahini dressing.

3. Garnish with fresh parsley if desired.

Cooking Time: Minimal (if using canned chickpeas).

9. Sardine and Avocado Toast

Ingredients:

- Sardines in olive oil
- Sliced avocado
- Gluten-free bread (toasted)
- Lemon juice and black pepper (for seasoning)

Instructions:

1. Toast the gluten-free bread.

2. Top with sliced avocado and sardines.

3. Drizzle with lemon juice and season with black pepper.

Cooking Time: Depends on bread toasting time.

10. Egg Salad Lettuce Wraps

Ingredients:

- Hard-boiled eggs (chopped)

- Diced celery and red onion
- Plain Greek yogurt (unsweetened)
- Dijon mustard (candida-friendly)
- Romaine lettuce leaves

Instructions:

1. In a bowl, mix chopped hard-boiled eggs, diced celery, and red onion.

2. Stir in plain Greek yogurt and Dijon mustard for creaminess and flavor.

3. Spoon the egg salad onto romaine lettuce leaves and wrap them up.

Cooking Time: Depends on egg boiling time.

CHAPTER FOUR

Candida Cleansing Dinner Recipes

Dinner is a crucial part of your candida cleansing journey. These dinner recipes are free of candida-promoting ingredients and focus on whole, unprocessed foods to support your digestive health.

1. Grilled Lemon Herb Chicken

Ingredients:

- Chicken breast or thigh fillets
- Fresh lemon juice
- Garlic (minced)
- Fresh herbs (such as rosemary and thyme)
- Olive oil
- Salt and pepper to taste

Instructions:

1. Marinate the chicken in lemon juice, minced garlic, fresh herbs, olive oil, salt, and pepper for at least 30 minutes.

2. Grill the chicken until fully cooked, turning occasionally.

3. Serve with a side of steamed vegetables or cauliflower rice.

Cooking Time: 15-20 minutes.

2. Baked Cod with Garlic Butter

Ingredients:

- Cod fillets
- Minced garlic
- Olive oil or ghee
- Fresh parsley (chopped)
- Lemon wedges
- Salt and pepper to taste

Instructions:

1. Preheat your oven to 375°F (190°C).

2. In an ovenproof dish, place the cod fillets.

3. Mix minced garlic, olive oil or ghee, fresh parsley, salt, and pepper. Drizzle this mixture over the cod.

4. Bake until the cod flakes easily with a fork.

5. Serve with lemon wedges and steamed vegetables.

Cooking Time: 15-20 minutes.

3. Cauliflower and Broccoli Soup

Ingredients:

- Cauliflower florets
- Broccoli florets
- Vegetable broth
- Onion (chopped)
- Garlic (minced)
- Olive oil
- Salt and pepper to taste

Instructions:

1. In a large pot, sauté chopped onion and minced garlic in olive oil until softened.

2. Add cauliflower and broccoli florets.

3. Pour in vegetable broth, cover, and simmer until vegetables are tender.

4. Use an immersion blender to puree the soup until smooth.

5. Season with salt and pepper to taste.

Cooking Time: 30-40 minutes.

4. Spaghetti Squash with Pesto

Ingredients:

- Spaghetti squash
- Candida-friendly pesto sauce
- Cherry tomatoes (halved)
- Pine nuts (toasted, optional)

Instructions:

1. Cut the spaghetti squash in half and remove the seeds.

2. Roast the squash halves in the oven until the flesh can be easily scraped into "noodles" with a fork.

3. Toss the spaghetti squash noodles with candida-friendly pesto sauce and halved cherry tomatoes.

4. Top with toasted pine nuts if desired.

Cooking Time: 45 minutes (mostly roasting time).

5. Lemon Herb Zucchini Noodles

Ingredients:

- Zucchini noodles (zoodles)
- Fresh lemon juice

- Fresh herbs (such as basil and parsley)
- Olive oil
- Garlic (minced)
- Salt and pepper to taste

Instructions:

1. In a pan, sauté minced garlic in olive oil until fragrant.

2. Add zucchini noodles and toss until tender.

3. Mix in fresh lemon juice, fresh herbs, salt, and pepper.

4. Serve as a light and refreshing side dish.

Cooking Time: 10 minutes.

6. Stuffed Bell Peppers

Ingredients:

- Bell peppers
- Ground turkey or chicken
- Cauliflower rice
- Diced tomatoes (canned, unsweetened)
- Onion and garlic (minced)
- Olive oil

- Italian seasoning

- Salt and pepper to taste

Instructions:

1. Cut the tops off bell peppers and remove seeds.

2. In a skillet, sauté minced onion and garlic in olive oil until softened.

3. Add ground turkey or chicken and cook until browned.

4. Mix in cauliflower rice, diced tomatoes, Italian seasoning, salt, and pepper.

5. Stuff the bell peppers with the mixture and bake until peppers are tender.

Cooking Time: 30-40 minutes.

7. Grilled Shrimp and Vegetable Skewers

Ingredients:

- Shrimp (peeled and deveined)

- Assorted vegetables (e.g., bell peppers, zucchini, cherry tomatoes)

- Olive oil

- Garlic (minced)

- Lemon juice

- Fresh herbs (such as basil and oregano)
- Salt and pepper to taste

Instructions:

1. Thread shrimp and assorted vegetables onto skewers.

2. In a bowl, mix olive oil, minced garlic, lemon juice, fresh herbs, salt, and pepper.

3. Brush the skewers with the olive oil mixture.

4. Grill until shrimp are pink and vegetables are tender.

5. Serve with a side salad.

Cooking Time: 15-20 minutes.

8. Turkey and Vegetable Stir-Fry

Ingredients:

- Ground turkey
- Assorted vegetables (e.g., bell peppers, broccoli, snap peas)
- Garlic and ginger (minced)
- Coconut aminos (for seasoning)
- Olive oil for stir-frying

-   Chopped scallions for garnish (optional)

Instructions:

1. Heat olive oil in a pan.

2. Add minced garlic and ginger and sauté until fragrant.

3. Add ground turkey and cook until browned.

4. Stir in assorted vegetables and cook until tender.

5. Season with coconut aminos and garnish with chopped scallions if desired.

Cooking Time: 20-25 minutes.

9. Baked Chicken Thighs with Roasted Vegetables

Ingredients:

-   Chicken thighs
-   Assorted vegetables (e.g., carrots, Brussels sprouts, sweet potatoes)
-   Olive oil
-   Herbs (such as rosemary and thyme)
-   Salt and pepper to taste

Instructions:

1. Preheat your oven to 375°F (190°C).

2. Place chicken thighs and assorted vegetables in a baking dish.

3. Drizzle with olive oil, season with herbs, salt, and pepper.

4. Bake until chicken is cooked through and vegetables are tender.

Cooking Time: 40-50 minutes.

10. Beef and Vegetable Stir-Fry

Ingredients:

- Thinly sliced beef strips
- Assorted vegetables (e.g., bell peppers, broccoli, snap peas)
- Garlic and ginger (minced)
- Coconut aminos (for seasoning)
- Olive oil for stir-frying
- Sesame seeds for garnish (optional)

Instructions:

1. Heat olive oil in a pan.

2. Sauté minced garlic and ginger until fragrant.

3. Add beef strips and cook until browned.

4. Stir in assorted vegetables and cook until tender.

5. Season with coconut aminos and garnish with sesame seeds if desired.

Cooking Time: 20-25 minutes.

Candida Cleansing Snacks Recipes

Snacking can be an enjoyable part of your candida cleansing journey. These snack recipes are free of candida-promoting ingredients and focus on whole, unprocessed foods to support your digestive health.

1. Guacamole with Veggie Sticks

Ingredients:

- Ripe avocados
- Lime juice
- Minced garlic

- Diced tomatoes
- Chopped cilantro
- Salt and pepper to taste
- Veggie sticks (carrots, cucumber, bell peppers) for dipping

Instructions:

1. Mash ripe avocados and mix with lime juice, minced garlic, diced tomatoes, and chopped cilantro.

2. Season with salt and pepper.

3. Serve with veggie sticks for dipping.

Preparation Time: 10 minutes.

2. Greek Yogurt with Berries

Ingredients:

- Unsweetened Greek yogurt
- Fresh berries (e.g., blueberries, strawberries, raspberries)
- A drizzle of honey (optional)
- Chopped nuts (e.g., almonds or walnuts) for crunch (optional)

Instructions:

1. In a bowl, spoon Greek yogurt.

2. Top with fresh berries.

3. Drizzle with honey for sweetness if desired.

4. Add chopped nuts for added texture.

Preparation Time: 5 minutes.

3. Cucumber and Hummus Slices

Ingredients:

- Cucumber slices
- Homemade or store-bought hummus (candida-friendly)

Instructions:

1. Slice cucumbers into rounds.

2. Serve with a side of hummus for dipping.

Preparation Time: 5 minutes.

4. Chia Seed Pudding

Ingredients:

- Chia seeds
- Unsweetened almond milk or coconut milk
- A drizzle of vanilla extract (candida-friendly)
- Fresh berries for topping

Instructions:

1. Mix chia seeds, almond milk or coconut milk, and vanilla extract in a bowl.

2. Stir well and refrigerate for at least 3 hours or overnight.

3. Top with fresh berries before serving.

Preparation Time: 3 hours (mostly resting time).

5. Sliced Bell Peppers with Almond Butter

Ingredients:

- Bell peppers (sliced)
- Almond butter (unsweetened)

Instructions:

1. Slice bell peppers into strips.

2. Dip in unsweetened almond butter for a crunchy, satisfying snack.

Preparation Time: 5 minutes.

6. Mixed Nuts and Seeds

Ingredients:

- A mix of unsalted nuts (e.g., almonds, walnuts, cashews) and seeds (e.g., pumpkin, sunflower)

Instructions:

1. Combine a variety of unsalted nuts and seeds in a snack-sized container.

2. Portion out for a satisfying, crunchy snack.

Preparation Time: Minimal (if using pre-packaged nuts and seeds).

7. Deviled Eggs

Ingredients:

- Hard-boiled eggs
- Homemade or store-bought mayonnaise (candida-friendly)
- Dijon mustard (candida-friendly)
- Paprika for garnish

Instructions:

1. Cut hard-boiled eggs in half.

2. Remove yolks and mix with mayonnaise and Dijon mustard.

3. Spoon the mixture back into the egg halves.

4. Garnish with paprika.

Preparation Time: Depends on egg boiling time.

8. Coconut Yogurt with Cinnamon

Ingredients:

- Unsweetened coconut yogurt
- Ground cinnamon

Instructions:

1. Spoon unsweetened coconut yogurt into a bowl.

2. Sprinkle with ground cinnamon for flavor.

Preparation Time: 2 minutes.

9. Sliced Apple with Almond Butter
Ingredients:

-   Apple slices
-   Unsweetened almond butter

Instructions:

1. Slice apples into rounds.

2. Spread with unsweetened almond butter for a satisfying, crunchy snack.

Preparation Time: 5 minutes.

10. Fermented Pickles
Ingredients:

-   Candida-friendly fermented pickles (e.g., sauerkraut, kimchi)
-   Cucumber slices (optional)

Instructions:

1. Enjoy a serving of fermented pickles or kimchi.

2. For extra crunch, serve with cucumber slices.

Preparation Time: Minimal.

CONCLUSION

The candida cleansing diet is a purposeful and systematic approach to addressing candida overgrowth in the body, a condition that can lead to a wide range of health issues if left unchecked. This dietary regimen emphasizes the elimination of candida-promoting foods while promoting the consumption of anti-fungal, nutrient-dense, and gut-friendly options. As we've explored in this guide, the diet primarily involves avoiding sugar, refined carbohydrates, processed foods, and alcohol, which are known to feed candida.

Throughout the cleansing process, individuals are encouraged to consume foods such as lean proteins, leafy greens, non-starchy vegetables, probiotic-rich fermented foods, nuts, seeds, and healthy fats. These choices provide essential nutrients, support a balanced gut microbiome, and help reduce inflammation, which is often associated with candida overgrowth.

One of the key benefits of the candida cleansing diet is its potential to alleviate a wide range of symptoms related to candida overgrowth, such as digestive discomfort, recurring yeast infections, fatigue, and brain fog. By restoring balance to the gut microbiota and reducing candida overgrowth, individuals may experience improved overall health and well-being.

However, it's important to note that the candida cleansing diet is not a one-size-fits-all solution, and its effectiveness can vary from person to person. It's essential to consult with a healthcare professional before embarking on any significant dietary changes, especially if you suspect candida overgrowth. They can help you determine whether a candida cleansing diet is appropriate for your specific health needs and provide guidance on its implementation.

In conclusion, the candida cleansing diet is a valuable tool for those seeking relief from candida-related health issues. When approached mindfully and with professional guidance, it can contribute to better gut health, improved vitality, and a reduced risk of candida overgrowth-related symptoms. Remember that every individual's journey is unique, and it's essential to prioritize long-term dietary and lifestyle changes to maintain a healthy balance in the gut and overall well-being